Agewell® Series on Health

Your Health is Our Biz™

New Medicine

Your Guide to Clinical Research

By Stephen A. Rappaport, M.D.

Published by Agewell®

International Standard Book Number: 1-886107-16-5

Published by Agewell®
9292 N. Meridian St. #107
Indianapolis, IN 46260

First Edition

RESEAÙ™ Resource
Puts the Accent on Ù™

The purpose of this book is to inform and educate. It is not a substitute for medical advice.

Contents

1

The Benefits of Medications

Medicines have transformed modern life and increased our life expectancy. One hundred years ago, people could expect to live an average of less than 50 years. But a child born today in the United States can expect to live over 76 years. Medicines are the result of scientific knowledge applied over a long period of time. They have prevented and cured disease, relieved pain and improved the quality of life.

Medicines have helped cut death from heart disease and stroke by nearly 50% over the past 30 years. Today we can control blood pressure, help prevent stroke, and decrease cholesterol and heart attacks. Improved medicines for arthritis decrease joint pain and disability with fewer side effects than ever before. Because of new treatments, cancer deaths have been falling continually over the past decade — most rapidly in recent years. Several new classes of drugs have vastly expanded the treatment of mood problems like depression.

Availability of medicines has motivated both doctors and patients to recognize and treat chronic conditions more effectively. These include problems such as osteoporosis, bladder weakness, decreased vision, and memory loss. Improved treatments allow senior adults today to live more active lives than previous generations.

Millions of people go to the pharmacy each day with prescriptions for drugs that they take for granted. Yet we have all benefited from the development of safe and effective treatments for numerous diseases — including some that have plagued humanity for thousands of years. In this chapter, we will look more closely at the process of scientific discovery that leads to the development of new medicines.

More people are actively seeking information about new medications and about how to use them appropriately. A flourishing health industry in the United States can provide us with an active flow of new treatment options. But individuals like us play a key role because we share in the development process through clinical trials – perhaps the most crucial part of clinical research. By knowing more about how drugs progress from laboratory to human, we can be aware of opportunities to participate in clinical trials. This ultimately benefits our community, our world, and us.

The Food and Drug Administration (FDA)

One hundred years ago, many actively promoted drugs were unsafe and ineffective. Our standards today are far greater. But to insure availability of high quality drugs that are safe and effective, there must be a way to keep ineffective or unsafe drugs off the market. This is largely the responsibility of a government agency called the **Food and Drug Administration (FDA)**. We start this overview of drug development by asking some fundamental questions:

WHAT IS THE FOOD AND DRUG ADMINISTRATION (FDA) AND WHAT DOES IT DO?

The FDA is a consumer protection agency within the Department of Health and Human Services (HHS). Its wide variety of responsibilities include insuring the safety of food, cosmetics, medical devices, and veterinary supplies. But of most interest to us is the FDA's best-known activity — overseeing drug evaluation and research. The FDA has responsibility for overseeing the safety and effectiveness of all types of drugs whether prescription, over-the-counter, or generic. The FDA is charged with preventing quackery. The agency also provides physicians and patients with essential information about appropriate use of medication. It oversees the research, development, manufacture and marketing of every drug and ensures that a drug's health benefits outweigh its risks.

DOES THE FDA TEST DRUGS?

The FDA does not develop, manufacture, or test drugs. The FDA analyzes extensive data that drug manufacturers submit in order to answer whether a particular drug works well for its proposed use. In short, the FDA determines if a drug can be approved based on its benefits and risks.

ARE FDA APPROVED DRUGS PERFECTLY SAFE?

No drug is "perfectly" safe. Every drug that affects the body can have potential side effects. The benefits of approved drugs outweigh the risks: thus in appropriate use, the side effects are not serious. The FDA also makes sure that the label in the package of every drug accurately outlines the benefits and risks determined through research.

Prescription, Over-the-Counter, and Generic Drugs

Certain drugs require a physician's order, but many are available without a prescription. Some drugs are only available from one manufacturer while others are made by several manufacturers. In this chapter, we will discuss these different kinds of drugs.

WHAT IS A **PRESCRIPTION** MEDICINE?

Prescription medicines are those prescribed and administered under supervision of a physician. They require a prescription or physician's authorization for purchase.

There are several reasons why some medicines may be sold only in this way:

- The disease or condition treated may be serious and require expertise for its management
- Different diseases can cause similar symptoms that only a physician can correctly differentiate and diagnose
- Medications may be dangerous if they are used for treatment of the wrong disease

WHAT ARE **OVER-THE-COUNTER** DRUGS?

Over-the-counter drugs are available to consumers without a doctor's prescription. Some drugs are initially approved for sale over-the-counter. More often, medications first approved as prescription drugs later switch to become over-the-counter drugs.

WHY ARE THERE MORE OVER-THE-COUNTER OR NON-PRESCRIPTION DRUGS THAN EVER BEFORE?

Many people today want to actively participate in their own healthcare and treatment decisions. To accommodate this trend, the FDA considers switching a drug from prescription to over-the-counter availability when this change will benefit consumers without endangering their safety. An important consideration is whether a person can reasonably self-diagnose and treat a certain condition. Many common ailments that range from skin problems to colds can be successfully diagnosed and treated without need for a physician.

WHAT ARE **GENERIC** DRUGS?

Generic drugs are medications chemically identical to those sold under a brand name. During the approval process the FDA compares a potential generic drug to the name-brand drug. The generic has to have the same active ingredient(s) and strength. It must also have the same dosage forms such as tablet, patch or liquid. A person must be able to take a generic medication the same way as the name brand, for example, by injecting it or swallowing it. The labeling on the generic must be similar. Finally, the generic must be "bioequivalent" to the name-brand drug; it must be proven to have a similar rate and extent of absorption, and it must be available to the same site in the body where it is needed.

Like all drugs, generics must meet standards of strength, quality, purity, and potency. But generic drugs can cost significantly less than prescription drugs; in this way, use of generics helps decrease overall health care costs. There is often active competition to manufacture a generic after a name-brand drug's patent expires. Ultimately, this encourages companies to keep finding new and better medicines and to improve on the treatments currently available.

HOW CAN YOU BE SURE THAT A GENERIC IS "BIOEQUIVALENT" TO THE NAME-BRAND DRUG?

Since clinical trials for name-brand drugs may involve thousands of patients, generics need not replicate this extensive research. The safety and effectiveness of the product is already well established after years of patient use. It would be unnecessary to repeat the research.

But a generic drug application must undergo scientifically rigorous tests and procedures to demonstrate that the drug is bioequivalent, that is, it performs in the same manner as the name brand. Much of the emphasis in testing concerns evaluating the amount of active drug ingredient in the bloodstream and available to target organ systems or tissues. Scientists measure this at specific time intervals after taking the drug.

DO BOTH PRESCRIPTION AND OVER-THE-COUNTER DRUGS HAVE GENERICS AVAILABLE?

Both prescription and over-the-counter drugs may have generic versions. For example, the medication ibuprofen was once available only by prescription. Years later, ibuprofen switched to non-prescription and became an over-the-counter drug. Today ibuprofen is one of the most commonly used generic analgesic medicines, but it is also sold under the brand name of Advil®.

The Process of Drug Development

Scientific research provides insight into the causes of many diseases. But research moves forward slowly — in small carefully planned steps. First, scientists carry out tests in cells and tissues called basic research. Some disease processes are complex — involving a sequence of biological events. Scientists break these events down into component parts and carefully analyze them. Research efforts then target the effects of a new medicine to correct the abnormal events occurring in the cells.

It may take years before this work yields promising leads. If this basic research is successful, testing continues in animals. Only after extensively studying outcomes of tests in animals, can clinical researchers begin to consider drug evaluation with people.

WHAT CLUES DO LABORATORY SCIENTISTS USE TO TARGET A POTENTIAL NEW DRUG?

Rarely, scientists find the right compound quickly or through luck. The process usually takes much more time than anticipated. Often thousands of compounds must be tested to find one that works. For example, scientists may add a potential drug little by little to an enzyme or a cell culture. They find which of these additions show the desired chemical effect. In recent years, researchers have used computers to simulate enzyme action and to design chemicals that might work in a particular situation. Research findings continually lead to changes in drug design or to more extensive experimentation. We will never know everything about the human body, so there is no end to the research process.

IS ANIMAL TESTING HUMANE? IS IT NECESSARY?

Scientists overseeing animal testing make deliberate efforts to use as few animals as possible and to make sure that the animals receive proper care. Because a particular drug may affect one species differently from another, testing may occur in different types of animals.

Animal tests are important because they show whether a potential drug has unacceptable side effects and how safe the drug is at different doses. These results are necessary to subsequently evaluate the way in which people can use a particular drug. Analyzing how a drug works is very tricky. There are effects of the drug on the body, but there are also effects of the body on the drug. The manner in which a drug is absorbed or broken down makes a big difference in treatment decisions.

WHAT KINDS OF SCIENTISTS DO DRUG RESEARCH?

Many different members make up the scientific teams that study new drugs. **Biochemists** are experts in the chemistry involved in life processes. **Molecular biologists** study molecules that make up living matter. **Toxicologists** investigate the potential for a new chemical to cause harm. **Pharmacologists** evaluate the mechanisms by which drugs work. **Computer scientists** are increasing involved in applying a high tech approach using sophisticated machines to analyze new chemicals. The process of drug discovery requires combining all of these different scientific perspectives in the overall effort.

IS DRUG DISCOVERY EXPENSIVE?

Drug discovery is extremely expensive. This is partly because of the rigorous scientific method used, but also because many seemingly promising drugs have to eventually be rejected. If a medicine is poorly absorbed or is unsafe before completion of animal testing — it will not be developed any further. Sometimes, drug doses may not prove effective enough.

There is careful consideration about when to discontinue research on a drug. In fact, a very small number of all drugs evaluated ever reach the point where they are suitable for testing in people.

Until the twentieth century, little was known about how drugs worked. There were no accepted scientific standards. Medicines sold often caused more harm than good. Prescribing and taking drugs was risky for physicians and patients alike.

Today we have a process of drug development and evaluation to make sure that new medicines are safe and effective. Sometimes people believe that our approval process for a new medicines takes too long when compared to other countries. It is not unusual for 10 years to pass from the time that an experimental drug is conceived in the laboratory to the time that it becomes available at the pharmacy. Crucial stages of drug development are the clinical trials that determine whether a drug is safe and effective, what doses are best, and what side effects occur. This information guides health professionals and consumer in proper use of medicines.

In the next chapter, we will look in greater detail at different types of clinical trials and their important roles in advancing our therapeutic options.

2

An Overview of Clinical Trials

Clinical research trials—in short, clinical trials— are research studies to test the safety and effectiveness of a new drug. They are the final step in the long process that begins with preliminary laboratory research and animal testing. These trials evaluate the potential clinical usefulness of a therapy or compare an investigational treatment against standard treatment. Each clinical trial answers specific questions to find better ways to prevent, detect, or treat diseases or to improve care.

Clinical trials are a critical part of the research process. They gradually help to move research from the laboratory to become widely available for many people. Clinical trials have resulted in enormous strides in finding new treatments for diseases.

WHO DEVELOPS THE IDEAS FOR CLINICAL TRIALS?

Some of the same experts from the team that tested new therapies in the laboratory and animal studies continue to participate; for example, chemists focus on the strength, quality and purity of the drug and pharmacologists evaluate the drug's effects. Other team members that take active roles include:

- Pharmacokinetic experts who evaluate the way the drug is made available to the body
- Statisticians who make sure accurate conclusions come from the design of the study
- Physicians who look at the drug's therapeutic and adverse effects
- Microbiologists who are experts in how an antibiotic drug affects microorganisms such as bacteria, viruses, and fungi.

Clinical trials answer specific questions about the effects of a drug or therapy to improve health. Planning for trials begins far in advance. They follow a rigorous scientific process that has built-in safeguards for participants. Clinical trials usually proceed in a series of steps called phases. Initially in the early phase, small trials test the safety of the drug. In later phases, larger trials test the effectiveness of the drug compared to current standards of care.

Based on the early research and preclinical testing, the sponsor of the clinical trial files an application for an Investigational New Drug with the FDA. After FDA experts approve the start of clinical trials, progressive phases of testing get under way. The process for gaining final approval of a drug involves three kinds of trials called Phase 1, Phase 2, and Phase 3. Each phase of research is designed to answer different types of questions.

WHAT IS THE PURPOSE OF A PHASE 1 CLINICAL TRIAL?

A phase 1 trial finds the best way to give people a new medicine, how often to give it, and what the safest dose is. There also are special laboratory and blood tests to evaluate how a new drug is working in the body.

WHAT HAPPENS IN A PHASE 1 TRIAL?

A phase 1 trial usually takes place only in few locations and enrolls a small number of patients. For example, a phase 1 trial may divide a group of less than 30 participants into subgroups of 3 to 6 people. In turn, each of these subgroups may receive a different dose of the new drug.

Because the initial dosing is based on the preclinical testing, the drug received is usually a very conservative amount. If evaluation of initial treatment shows safety, a group of participants may receive a bit more drug. This pattern continues with close and careful oversight.

There are some special variations of Phase 1 trials, for example:

- Evaluating new doses or combinations of established drugs
- Focusing on older adults if other trials have only young people

WHAT IS THE PURPOSE OF A PHASE 2 CLINICAL TRIAL?

A phase 2 trial continues to test the safety of the new medicine and evaluate how well it works for a more specific condition.

WHAT HAPPENS IN A PHASE 2 TRIAL?

While Phase 1 trials may involve only 20 to 80 people, Phase 2 trials look at the effectiveness of a drug in a larger group — perhaps 100 to 300 participants. Using the dosage determined in phase 1 trials, phase 2 trials often focus more specifically on certain aspects of a disease.

All participants in a phase 2 trial receive the same intervention — often the same dose of a drug. Sometimes, phase 2 trials compare different doses of a drug, or different times of the day to take it. The phase 2 research provides important additional information about effectiveness and safety.

But certain key questions remain that phase 2 trials cannot answer. Phase 2 trials are often relatively short, so further clinical trials must determine a drug's long-term benefits. Phase 2 trials usually do not compare a drug to other therapy, so subsequent larger trials must establish the true value of the treatment. For these reasons, promising drugs continue for Phase 3 clinical trials.

WHAT IS THE PURPOSE OF A PHASE 3 CLINICAL TRIAL?

Phase 3 trials compare the new treatment to a standard treatment. Phase 3 questions focus on how well a new drug compares to the most widely accepted treatment. The purpose is to see whether the new treatment is better than, the same as, or not as good as the standard treatment.

WHAT HAPPENS DURING A PHASE 3 TRIAL?

Phase 3 trials are larger than Phase 2. There may be 1000 to 4000 or more participants. Phase 3 studies have these main goals:

- Confirming the effectiveness of a drug
- Monitoring the side effects
- Showing the medical importance of the results.

Like Phase 2 trials, Phase 3 trials usually focus on specific types of disease. Participants are assigned at random to a group that is given the new treatment or to a group that receives the standard treatment. If there is no standard treatment, a phase 3 trial may include treatment with a medicine designed to look like the test medicine but without any active ingredient. We will discuss the use of a "placebo" — sometimes called a "sugar pill" — in the next chapter. Phase 3 trials usually occur at many sites around the country. Because these trials guide health professionals in treatment decisions, they may include measures of function and quality of life.

When analysis of the Phase 3 trial is complete, researchers will carefully evaluate the data. Usually they will inform the medical community of the results in scientific journals or at conferences. But if trial results have significant medical importance, there may be a public announcement soon afterward to make sure that many people can benefit quickly from the advance. Newspapers and television regularly feature such results. Once the drug is proven safe and effective, it may become the new standard of practice for physicians.

WHAT RESEARCH CONTINUES AFTER THE PHASE 3
TRIAL?

Phase 4 trials look even more closely at a drug's long-term safety and effectiveness. Because these occur after the FDA has already approved a drug for use, phase 4 trials are sometimes referred to as **post-clinical** trials. Phase 4 trials are not as common as phase 1, phase 2, or phase 3 trials. But they often have a significant influence on medical practice because hundreds or even thousands of people participate.

Summary

This chapter has discussed the four phases of clinical trials including their purposes and differing designs. Let's briefly review each phase to compare the main questions that clinical trials address:

Phase 1 trials evaluate:
- How does the treatment affect the human body?
- How should the treatment be given?
- What dosage is safe?

Phase 2 trials evaluate:
- Does the treatment do what it is supposed to do for a particular disease?
- How does the treatment affect the human body?

Phase 3 trials evaluate:

- Is the new treatment better than current practice?

Phase 4 trials evaluate:

- What are the effects of an approved treatment?

In the next chapter, will look more closely at the specific design of a clinical trial using its structural "blueprint" called the **protocol.**

3

Participation in
a Protocol

Purposes

Clinical trials may have four different purposes:

- **Prevention** trials seek to prevent disease or reduce the chance of developing it; the trials often involve healthy people.
- **Screening** trials are designed to detect a disease before it causes symptoms.
- **Diagnostic** trials look at tests or procedures to identify a disease more accurately at an earlier stage.
- **Treatment** trials treat a condition or improve the quality of life.

Treatment trials systematically evaluate quality of life. They look at a variety of innovations including interventions to improve the comfort and well-being of people especially those with a particular condition or disease.

Some research involves innovative surgical procedures or new devices like blood glucose monitors. But this book focuses primarily on treatment trials whose purpose is to evaluate drugs or combinations of drugs by asking:

- What new treatment approaches can help people?
- What is the most effective treatment for people?

All clinical trials involve scientific approach, but they differ by type and phase. Trials follow strict guidelines according to the study design. A trial usually has a physician in charge called the principal investigator. There are specific criteria about which people will be able to participate.

The Protocol

The principal investigator's plan for a study – called a **protocol** — is more detailed than a recipe. It describes the background of the study, objectives, and the design, setup, and organization. Each center participating in a clinical trial uses the same protocol. This ensures consistency of procedures and improved communication. The standardization and uniformity allow the results from all centers to be combined and compared when they are analyzed.

Required Protocol Elements

- General information
- Background information (references from the scientific literature)
- Trial objectives and purpose
- Trial design
- Participant selection and withdrawal
- Participant treatment
- Efficacy assessment
- Safety assessment
- Statistics
- Direct access to source data and documents
- Quality control and quality assurance
- Ethics
- Data handling and record keeping

The protocol specifies the reasons for doing a study:

- What is the basis for conducting a trial?
- What is the scientific rationale?
- What are the objectives?

The protocol contains information about people who can participate in the study:

- How many participants?
- Who is eligible to participate based on health?

The protocol describes in detail what medication participants will take, the dosage and frequency:

- What is the intervention?
- How long does it last?
- How often is it given?
- What dose effect might occur?

Finally, the protocol specifies information about data collection:

- What medical tests will participants have? How often?
- What information will be gathered?
- What are the endpoints of the study?

Working Together

Clinical trials can appear complex and confusing. But most are organized in a very logical manner. The best way to guide you through the pathway is a sequential question and answer format. Developing a new medication requires several different parties to work together. We begin with a more detailed look at these parties, their roles, and their interactions:

- Sponsor
- Participant
- Research team
- Ethical review board — often called an Institutional Review Board (IRB).

The Sponsor

WHAT DOES A SPONSOR DO?

Sponsors are the agents responsible for organizing, overseeing, and funding a clinical trial. Pharmaceutical companies often sponsor clinical trials as well as private organizations like the American Heart Association. Federal agencies such as the National Institutes of Health (NIH), the Department of Defense, and the Department of Veteran's Affairs (VA) have active clinical research programs.

WHO PAYS FOR THE COSTS ASSOCIATED WITH A CLINICAL TRIAL?

Sponsors usually pay for the patient care costs such as drugs, physician visits, and lab tests associated with a clinical trial. If enough data show that a treatment approach is safe and effective, a health plan may consider covering some or all of the costs.

WHERE DO CLINICAL TRIALS TAKE PLACE?

In previous years, clinical trials were conducted primarily at medical centers. Increasingly, they take place in a variety of locations including physician offices, clinics, or hospitals.

The Principal Investigator and Clinical Trial Coordinator

The essence of a clinical trial can be described very simply. A research team of health care professionals:

- Checks the health of the participant at the beginning of the trial
- Gives specific instructions about how to participate in the trial
- Monitors the participant carefully during the trials
- Stays in touch after the trial is completed.

Participants in a clinical trial work with the different members of the research team. It is helpful for us to look more closely at the work of different team members.

WHAT DOES THE PRINCIPAL INVESTIGATOR DO?

The principal investigator, usually a physician, conducts the clinical trial. In addition to overseeing the treatment, the principal investigator has a variety of other responsibilities:

- Concept development
- Protocol writing
- Institutional review board submission
- Working with potential participants
- Overseeing informed consent of all participants
- Data collection and analysis.

WHAT DOES THE CLINICAL TRIAL COORDINATOR DO?

A clinical trial coordinator, usually a nurse, has a major role in operations of the project. The coordinator assists in giving information about the project and obtaining consent. Above all, the coordinator:

- Monitors for responses to treatment
- Checks for problems or side effects of treatment
- Manages and analyzes data
- Ensures quality in the trial and that operations proceed according to the protocol.

The clinical trial coordinator makes sure the principal investigator has sufficient information to make the best decisions throughout the course of the trial. The coordinator also maintains communication with the other team members, clinical trial participants, and other doctors who have referred patients for the project.

The Participants

WHO CAN PARTICIPATE IN A CLINICAL TRIAL?

Participants are the most critical people involved in a clinical trial. The protocol of every clinical trial clearly states the types of people who can or cannot participate. This helps ensure safety of participants; for example, some potential participants have additional health problems that could be made worse by the treatment in a study. All potential participants interested in a clinical trial receive medical tests in the beginning to be sure that no one with special risks joins the study.

Participant selection is necessary for a trial to yield accurate and meaningful results. For this reason, trials sometimes will exclude individuals who have previously had specific kinds of treatment. With such requirements, researchers can have confidence that a participant's results are due to study treatment and not to earlier treatments received.

HOW SPECIFIC ARE ELIGIBILITY CRITERIA?

Participant eligibility criteria may generally specify about age, sex, or type of disease. They may have detailed restrictions, for example, about prior treatments, blood cell counts, electrocardiogram findings, or function of organ systems. Eligibility criteria may vary depending upon the phase of the trial. In phase 1 and phase 2, the entry criteria usually have a goal of ensuring that people with abnormal organ function are not put at risk. By the time phase 3 trials are ready to begin, much more is known about a drug so that these trials may have more precise requirements about disease type and prior treatments.

IF ELIGIBILITY CRITERIA ARE NARROW, WILL MANY POTENTIAL PARTICIPANTS FAIL TO QUALIFY?

Clinical trials attempt to include as many types of people as possible. But if the criteria are too diverse, researchers may miss key groups of people that could benefit the most from treatment. A more diverse group of participants generally provides results that are useful for the population at large. In phase 3 trials, widely applicable results are desirable because they will benefit the maximum number of people.

The Institutional Review Board (IRB)

By following strict scientific guidelines, clinical trials protect people and provide sound results. These can lead to effective therapies. Experts from different disciplines review protocols for merit, value, and technique. Important issues they evaluate include:

1) **Significance**: Does the clinical trial address an important problem? How will it advance scientific

knowledge? What effect will the clinical trial have on current methods of treatment?

2) **Approach**: Are the design, methods, and analyses appropriate and developed enough? Have potential problems and alternatives been considered?

3) **Innovation**: Does the project include new concepts and methods? Is it original? Does the project challenge the way people do things now?

4) **Investigator**: Do the principal investigator and other researchers have the training and experience to carry out the project?

5) **Environment**: Does the project take place in a setting that contributes to its successful completion?

Many safeguards exist for participants in clinical trials. The sponsor and principal investigator have responsibilities for good trial design and operations. Participants also have an important role in ensuring safeguards. Later in the book, we discuss the **informed consent** process by which individuals learn details about the trial and decide whether or not to participate. But a specifically designated group called the **Institutional Review Board (IRB)** has responsibility for protection of clinical trial participants.

WHAT IS AN INSTITUTIONAL REVIEW BOARD (IRB)?

An IRB is a group of people from diverse occupations and backgrounds who continually review biomedical research involving people. The IRB's primacy purpose is to guarantee protection of participants' rights and welfare. IRBs are usually made up of various medical specialists, lay members from the community, and professionals such as ministers or attorneys. The people who serve on an IRB must be qualified to evaluate new and ongoing clinical trials on the basis of scientific, legal, and ethical merits.

Together, members of the board determine if the risks involved in a trial are reasonable with respect to the potential benefits. The IRB monitors the progress of a clinical trial from beginning to end.

WHAT DOES AN IRB DO?

IRBs have two main categories of responsibility: initial review of a clinical trial protocol and continuing review of trial operations. IRBs review and approve a research plan before the research is carried out. This review includes the protocol, the informed consent document to be signed by participants, and promotional materials for the project. The continuing review process is multifaceted and examines:

- changes or amendments to the clinical trial before they occur
- interval progress reports required throughout the trial
- unexpected experiences of trial participants to ensure that the risk to benefit ratio of the research remains acceptable.

WHAT ETHICAL PRINCIPLES GUIDE THE IRB'S WORK?

Three major principles underlie the viewpoint of an IRB:

- Respect for people – recognition of the personal dignity and autonomy of individuals and special protection for children, older adults, people with low education, and those with mental disabilities
- Protection from harm – maximizing benefits and minimizing risk of harm
- Justice – distributing research benefits and burdens fairly.

DOES AN IRB APPLY THESE PRINCIPLES TO CLINICAL TRIALS?

Yes. The first principle of medicine is doing no harm. Fully informed patients can consent to take part in a clinical trial that is controlled, randomized, and blinded—even when effective therapy exists—as long as this does not cause harm or irreversible injury.

Remember that most clinical trials have several major levels of review to protect all participants. This is true whether a trial takes place at a doctor's office of a hospital. Even after an IRB grants approval, the board continues to review the trial while it is underway. The frequency of review depends on the degree of risk involved. All trials have reviews at periodic intervals of:

- How many people are enrolled in a trial
- How many people have withdrawn
- Participants' experiences
- Progress to date.

Based on this information, the IRB decides whether the trial should continue as described in the original research plan. If not, the board tells the research team what changes must be made. If a research team does not follow these requirements or if evidence of unexpected harm emerges, the IRB can stop a clinical trial at any time.

When a principal investigator submits an application for a clinical trial, what does the IRB look for in the initial review?

The board ensures that risks to participants are minimized as much as possible through sound research design. Any risks must be reasonable in relation to the anticipated benefits. There must be equitable selection of participants. The informed consent document needs to be complete and clearly written. Collected data must be monitored in a way that insures participants' safety and protects privacy. IRBs require data confidentiality. The also make sure that any advertising is accurate.

The final vote on approval of a clinical trial includes different kinds of board members. Some are scientific experts; others purposely come from areas outside of science or health care. Some members are purposely not affiliated with the institution where the research will take place.

HOW LONG AGO WERE IRBS ESTABLISHED?

Public awareness and concern grew regarding the need for ethical review of clinical trials. The FDA regulations regarding IRBs were issued in 1981.

WHERE ARE IRBS LOCATED?

Over 1000 IRBs exist throughout the United States. Hospitals, medical schools, and government agencies that conduct research commonly have their own. Some managed care organizations also have an IRB. Some major IRBs exist independently of any institutions in which the research takes place.

WHO MAKES SURE THAT AN IRB IS DOING ITS WORK CORRECTLY?

Within the Department of Health and Human Services, The National Institutes of Health and the Food and Drug Administrationshare responsibility for IRBs. The FDA oversees records and operations to make sure that IRB approvals,safeguards, members, and operations are what they should be. The FDA requires the IRBs to submit specific information at intervals about their operations.

The Data and Safety Monitoring Board

Phase 3 trials often have a separate Data and Safety Monitoring Board (DSMB) that evaluates preliminary outcomes and other results during the trial. Made up of experts — including physicians, scientists, and statisticians — this board looks at all trial results to insure that any risks of participation are minimized to the extent possible. The DSMB can also stop a trial if safety concerns arise. If early results show clear advantages of a new drug, the DSMB may recommend ending the trial early and encourage wider user of the drug. On the other hand, if early results show an unforeseen negative effect, the trial is stopped immediately.

The IRB, DSMB, and FDA complement one another. They provide a system of checks and balances that help safeguard clinical trials. But these are no substitute for the most important element – an informed participant.

We have looked at the roles and responsibilities of the main parties involved in carrying out a clinical trial including the sponsor, principal investigator, clinical trial coordinator, and institutional review board.

With our knowledge of the people involved, we can overview the key issues in the structure of a clinical trial.

Clinical Trial Design

HOW LARGE ARE CLINICAL TRIALS?

Clinical trials must be sufficiently large to generate enough information to draw a valid conclusion; otherwise, important results may be missed. On the other hand, an unnecessarily large trial may take much too long to complete. The number of participants is very important. Experts in statistics advise the research team based on how large a difference would be medically important. With this understanding, statisticians can calculate how many people need to enter the trial for the results to be most useful.

Many clinical trials have three key elements in their design. These are especially common in phase 3 trials:

- Controlled
- Randomized
- Blinded.

WHAT DOES A **CONTROLLED** TRIAL MEAN?

In a controlled trial, there are two groups of participants. Those in the **investigational group** receive the new agent, treatment, or experimental drug being tested. The other participants in the **control group** receive a standard treatment for the disease. Standard treatment refers to the accepted, widely used treatment for a certain disease or condition.

The structure of an investigational group versus a control group is the standard way to design a trial in order to obtain observations that can be evaluated.

IS STANDARD TREATMENT EVER A "SUGAR PILL" OR PLACEBO?

In some cases, the control group may receive a placebo – which is an inactive pill, liquid or powder that has no treatment value. When the effectiveness of a new treatment may not be readily distinguished from established therapy, the only way to prove the benefit is to compare results against a placebo.

Even though a placebo contains an inactive substance, placebo treatment may still result in significant physical or emotional changes for the participant. These changes, called the placebo effect, are real and often beneficial, but they do not result from any special property of the substance. The improvement is due to the expectations of both the participant and of the treatment team.

WHAT IS A RANDOMIZED TRIAL?

Some phase 2 and most phase 3 trials are randomized. Randomization is a method that helps prevent bias in research. In a randomized trial, entering participants are assigned by chance either to a control group or an experimental therapy group. Neither the participants nor the physicians choose which treatment they receive.

WHY IS RANDOMIZATION IMPORTANT?

If either physicians or participants determined which therapy a participant would receive, there could be an unconscious bias in their assignments. In that case, bias would either make a treatment look more effective or less effective than it really is. Randomization produces groups with comparable characteristics that affect outcome. In this way, it helps guarantee that conclusions regarding effectiveness of a treatment are valid.

WHAT IS A BLINDED TRIAL?

A trial in which participants do not know which treatment they are receiving is called a **single-blinded** trial. A trial in which neither research team members nor participants know who is in the investigational or control group is called a **double-blinded** trial.

Double-blinded trial design ensures that people assessing the outcome of a project will not be influenced by knowledge of which intervention a participant is receiving. This makes the results of the clinical trial more reliable.

HAVEN'T SOME VERY IMPORTANT THERAPIES BEEN DISCOVERED WITHOUT THESE COMPLEX CLINICAL TRIALS?

The basics of a research program may seem straightforward. Recruit groups of people to participate, administer the drug to those who agree to take part, and see if it helps them. Some important treatments actually developed this way—for example, the rabies vaccine Louis Pasteur discovered in the 19th century. Rabies was always a fatal disease, and everyone who received the vaccine survived. The treatment was obviously proved effective. But this is an exceptional case. Most drugs are not miraculous cures for fatal diseases. They may relieve symptoms of an illness such as pain. A drug may reduce blood pressure or lower cholesterol to provide benefits over time. Effects like these can be more difficult to detect and evaluate.

In other cases, the measures of disease symptoms are subjective. For example, improvement of anxiety relies on the physician or patient interpretation. Expectation and hopes can influence these measurements. It becomes difficult to tell whether treatment has a favorable effect, no effect or even an adverse effect.

4

Personal Considerations

Taking Charge of Your Health

Clinical trials that are well designed and carried out are excellent ways for you to:

- Play an active role in your own health care
- Gain access to promising new approaches before they are widely available
- Obtain expert medical care and careful attention from a research team of health care professionals
- Help others in the future by contributing to medical research.

If you are interested in participating in a clinical trial, discuss the idea with your personal physician. The physician is often aware of and has access to information about investigational drugs that might be of benefit to you. A clinical trial may be conducted at a research center, but you often continue to work with your primary physician during the trial and after its completion.

Although clinical trials vary widely, you can expect some things in virtually all trials. You might have to give blood samples more often than you ordinarily would. You may be asked to undergo more frequent tests to assess your condition. Sometimes you may need to keep detailed records of your symptoms for review by the research team during the next visit.

The Informed Consent Process

Participation in a clinical trial does not guarantee that you will receive the investigational drug. But if there are control patients who might get a placebo, a research team member involved in the trial will explain this to you in advance. You will have to agree to the conditions of a clinical trial before participating. In this chapter, we will talk specifically about how to prepare for your meeting with the research team and what to expect during the informed consent process.

Participation in a research study involves understanding your potential risks and benefits as well as your rights and responsibilities. Informed consent is a process that provides you with explanations to make reasoned decisions about whether to begin or continue participating in a clinical trial. A written document alone does not guarantee that you fully understand what your participation means. So before you decide, a member of the research team will discuss with you the purpose of the trial, procedures, risk and potential benefits, and your rights as a participant. If you decide to participate, the team will continue to update you during the trial about any new information that may affect your participation. You will have opportunities to ask questions and raise concerns before, during and even after a trial

Remember that informed consent is an interactive, ongoing process, not a one-time information session.

Preparing for Participation

How well you and the research team communicate is one the most important parts of a good experience. This is not always easy; taking an active role in communication is a joint effort that requires time and effort from both sides. A good clinical research relationship is a partnership where the participant and team members work together to solve problems. This means you need to ask questions if explanations or instructions are unclear. Bring up problems even if someone doesn't ask first. Let a research team member know when a treatment is not working.

HOW CAN I GET READY FOR AN INITIAL MEETING WITH THE RESEARCH PHYSICIAN OR COORDINATOR?

Prepare a list of your concerns. Before going to the first visit, write down what you want to discuss. If you have more than a few items, put them in order so you are sure to ask about the most important ones first. Take along any information the research team may need such as your medical records and the names of your other doctors.

Fully inform the research team member you meet about your medical condition to make sure that a particular clinical trial is appropriate for you. Do not just say what you think someone wants to hear. Be honest about habits like smoking or about how closely you follow a special diet.

Bring a list of your medications. If you take several medicines, it is possible to have an interaction with the investigational drug. This can sometimes cause dangerous side effects. The research team member needs to know all of the medicines you take including non-prescription drugs, eye drops, vitamins, and laxatives. Describe how often you take each one and any drug allergies or reactions you have had.

Sometimes it is helpful to bring a family member or close friend with you. Let the person know in advance what the visit is about. The friend or relative can help remind you about what you planned to discuss and help in remembering the answers.

The initial meeting with a research team member begins the **process** of informed consent. This is a critical aspect of ensuring your safety in the trial. One of the main purposes of the meeting is for the team member to explain the trial in understandable language including:

- How the study is set up
- Possible risks and benefits
- Participation and medical care
- Your personal concerns.

Before looking at a model informed consent document, the next several pages provide a **checklist of questions to**

ask the research team. Each checklist outlines many likely areas of your concern. You can use the checklists as an aid to help you understand while you read through the document itself.

There is space on each page to write down comments. Your notes can provide a ready reference in your own words that will be helpful during the consent discussion and for future reference.

Immediately following the checklists, we will continue by examining the information covered in an informed consent document in greater detail.

A Checklist of Questions to Ask the Research Team

The Study

1. What is the purpose of the study?
2. Why do researchers think the approach may be effective?
3. Who will sponsor the study?
4. Who has reviewed and approved the study?
5. How are study results and safety of participants being checked?
6. How long will the study last?
7. What will be my responsibilities if I participate?
8. Who will answer questions I have during and after the trial?
9. What steps will be taken to protect my privacy and the confidentiality of my medical records?

Notes

A Checklist of Questions to Ask the Research Team

Benefits and Risks

1. What are my possible short-term benefits?
2. What are my possible long-term benefits?
3. What are my short-term risks, such as side effects?
4. What are my possible long-term risks?
5. What other options do I have?
6. How do the possible risks and benefits of this trial compare with those options?

Notes

A Checklist of Questions to Ask the Research Team

My Participation and Care

1. What kinds of therapies, procedures and tests will I have during the trial?
2. Will they hurt?
3. Will I be able to take my regular medications while in the trial?
4. Where will I receive medical care?
5. Will I have to be hospitalized?
6. Who will be in charge of my care?
7. What type of follow-up care is part of the study?

Notes

A Checklist of Questions to Ask the Research Team

Personal Concerns

1. How could participation in the study affect my daily life?
2. Can I talk to other people in the study?
3. Will I have to pay for any part of the trial such as tests or the study drug?
4. What is my health insurance likely to cover?
5. Who can help answer any questions that arise?
6. Will there be travel costs that I need to consider while I am in the trial?

Notes

The Informed Consent Document

Descriptive summaries of answers to the checklist questions appear in the **informed consent document**. Like any other medical procedure, a clinical trial has a written consent form. You may already have experience with signing a consent form if you have ever had surgery or hospital procedures. The informed consent document gives a summary of the trial's purpose and procedures, and it describes your rights.

TITLE

The first section of the document is the title. Read it carefully because the title is often very exact and descriptive. Each of the following sections of the informed consent document answers the main question that appears in bold print.

PURPOSE
Why is this clinical trial being done?

This section explains why researchers are conducting the trial:

- Because they have not found an effective treatment for a certain condition
- Because they are not sure which treatment method works best.

Remember the 3 different phases of a clinical trial that we discussed earlier:

Phase 1 trials test the safety and effectiveness of a new treatment or try to find the safe dose of a new drug.

Phase 2 trials evaluate the effects of a new treatment.

Phase 3 trials compare the effectiveness of a new treatment or treatment combination with that of standard treatment.

DESCRIPTION OF PROCEDURES
What is involved in the trial?

This section describes:
- The procedures that you will undergo
- How frequently you will have them
- Where they will take place (home, hospital, clinical center, or office

If the clinical trial is randomized, you will be assigned by computer into a study group. People in different groups will receive different treatments or treatment combinations so that researchers can evaluate which is most effective.

The informed consent document should make clear what procedures each of these groups will undergo. It should also indicate what your chances are of being placed in any one group.

DURATION
How long will I be in the trial?

This section describes:

- How long the trial will last
- Whether the trial involves follow-up, and if so, for how long.

This section also includes information about any circumstances under which the you should not continue the trial, for example if:

- If your health changes
- If new information indicates that it is best for you not to continue.

The informed consent document should make clear that you have the right to stop participating at any time. It should describe any possible medical consequences of sudden withdrawal.

RISKS
What are the risks of the trial?

This section describes the foreseeable physical risks such as side effects and indicates:

- Likelihood of these risks occurring
- How serious they may be
- Whether they are likely to be short-term (only during the trial)
- Whether they can possibly be long-term (weeks, months, or years after the trial).

The informed consent document should include specific information about reproductive risks, for example, whether you can nurse a child during the trial.

BENEFITS
What are the benefits of taking part?

The document describes any expected benefits for you or for others. A trial may or may not involve direct medical benefits to you, but it might lead to new knowledge that can help others in the future.

ALTERNATIVES
What are my options if I don't participate?

For treatment trials, this section describes what health care options you have besides participating in the trial. These often include other commonly used therapies.

CONFIDENTIALITY

This statement describes how your information will be kept confidential. It should explain that certain groups like the trial sponsor or government agencies like the FDA may have access to your records for quality assurance and data analysis.

ADDITIONAL EXPENSES

What are the costs?

This section indicates whether participating in the trial will result in added costs to you or your insurance company. It also covers other cost issues such as:

- Who will pay for emergency medical treatment in case of injury or illness
- Whether you will have to pay for drugs that become commercially available during the trial
- Whether or not you will receive payment for participating.

PARTICIPANT'S RIGHTS

What are my rights as a participant?

The document should specify that:

- Your participation is voluntary
- You can choose not to take part or leave at any time without penalty
- You will receive any new information that might affect your participation.

CONTACT INFORMATION

What if I have questions or problems?

You should have the name and phone number of a research team member to contact for questions related to the study or unforeseen problems that occur. You should also receive a phone number for the Institutional Review Board in case you have questions about your rights as a research participant.

THE SIGNATURE
Your legal consent to participate in the trial

Remember that the most important part of your initial visit with a research team member is not the informed consent **document** but the informed consent **process**. The heart of the informed consent process is your ongoing interaction and discussion with the research team.

Sometimes you may have a limited amount of time together. Make the best use of it by knowing what your most important questions are. Take along a note pad to write down the main points. Ask about information that is not clear at any visit during the trial. You may say, for example, "I want to make sure I understand. Could you explain that a little further?"

Share your point of view. It can be very difficult to absorb all of the information about a clinical trial in one sitting or when you first receive the informed consent document. If you feel rushed, you may say, "I'm really worried about this. I'd feel much better if we could talk about it a little more." You can take your copy of the informed consent document home. Review it as many times as you need, and discuss it with family and friends. Physicians and health professionals can be valuable sources of advice, but only you can make the decision about whether or not to participate.

New Information and Protocol Updates

The team member working with you should take steps to ensure your understanding of these basic issues:

- How each team member interacts with you
- Tests and procedures during the clinical trial
- Whom to contact about health or medication problems that occur
- Continuing updates on new information that could affect your health or desire to remain in the study.

Depending on the type of new information that becomes known during the course of the clinical trial, you may be contacted about signing a new and revised informed consent document.

Closing Thoughts

We have covered a great deal of information in this book. Review it at your own pace. Apply the principles discussed here to avoid misperceptions about a clinical trial and your participation in it. Consider using the checklists in this chapter as an aid to understanding the informed consent document. Good communication on both sides will help enhance the entire process.

I hope that a greater knowledge about clinical trials can help resolve unnecessary fears and open a chance to benefit from a new drug in the future.

A major polling organization recently conducted a study about the experiences of clinical trial participants. The overwhelming majority reported very positive feelings. By using this book for improved understanding and preparation, your clinical trial experience can be equally enriching.

Appendixes

Ethical Principles of the Belmont Report

Six Simple Suggestions for Success in a Study

Ethical Principles of the Belmont Report

The Belmont Report— published in 1979 – has greatly influenced current laws about research with people. Its three principles carry strong moral force and provide a comprehensive framework for ethical decision-making.

Virtually all clinical research professionals believe that it is important to understand and apply these principles:

1. Respect for Persons

This principle is based on the dignity and autonomy of individuals. It requires that participants in research give their informed consent. It also requires that certain groups of people — such as children, the mentally disabled, and the severely ill — need special protections because of their vulnerability.

2. Beneficence

This principle requires protection for all individuals by carefully designing clinical trials to maximize anticipated benefits and minimize possible harms. If the expected benefits do not justify the research risks – we must identify alternative ways to obtain the benefits.

3. Justice

This principle requires that we treat research participants fairly. The choice of participants should be equitable — including individuals from all groups likely to benefit from applications of the research. This principle also provides that groups unlikely to benefit from the research should not be included.

Six Simple Suggestions for Success with a Study

1. Learn the facts.

Before you decide to participate, learn and understand as much about the study as you can. Use the checklists in this book.

2. Speak up.

The more information your research team members know about you and your health, the better they can share relevant information about the clinical trial.

3. Ask questions.

The research team members can help you make informed choices, but you have to ask the right questions. When you meet with a team member, have your questions written down and take notes. Bring along a friend or relative to help you understand and remember the answers.

4. Balance benefits and risks.

After you have exchanged information, weigh your options. At a certain point, you must decide if the benefits of the clinical trial outweigh the risks. The final choice is yours.

5. Follow directions.

Follow directions from the research team throughout the course of the clinical trial. Take the doses exactly as prescribed. Read labels carefully.

6. Report back to the research team.

Pay attention to how you feel. Let a research team member know about any problems. If you experience a side effect, notify your contact person immediately.

Glossary

Adverse Event: An unwanted effect caused by the administration of drugs. Onset may be sudden or develop over time.

Approved Drugs: In the U.S., the Food and Drug Administration (FDA) must approve a substance as a drug before it can be marketed. The approval process involves several steps including pre-clinical laboratory and animal studies, clinical trials for safety and efficacy, filing of a New Drug Application by the manufacturer of the drug, FDA review of the application, and FDA approval/rejection of application.

Bias: Human choices, beliefs, or any other factors besides those being studied that affect a clinical trial's results. Clinical trials use many methods to avoid bias because biased results may not be correct.

Data and Safety Monitoring Board (DSMB): An independent committee composed of community representatives and clinical research experts. Responsibilities of the DSMB are to ensure that risks associated with participation are minimized to the extent possible, and stop a trial either if safety concerns arise or as soon as its objectives have been met.

Dose: The amount of drug administered to a patient or test participant at a single time.

Effectiveness: The desired measure of a drug's influence on a disease condition. Effectiveness must be proven by substantial evidence consisting of adequate and well-controlled investigations, including human studies by qualified experts, that prove the drug will have the effect claimed in its labeling.

Food and Drug Administration (FDA): An agency of the U.S. Department of Health and Human Services whose mission it is to promote and protect the public health: 1) by ensuring that medical products are proven safe and effective before they can be used by patients and 2) by monitoring products for continued safety after they are in use.

Hypothesis: A supposition or assumption advanced as a guide to experimental investigation.

Informed Consent Document: A document that describes the rights of the study participants, and includes details about the study, such as its purpose, duration, required procedures, and key contacts. Risks and potential benefits are explained in the informed consent document. The participant then decides whether or not to sign the document. Informed consent is not a contract and the participant may withdraw from the trial at any time.

Informed Consent: The process of providing all relevant information about the trial's purpose, risks, benefits, alternatives, and procedures to a potential participant, who then, consistent with his or her own interests and circumstances, makes an informed decision about whether to participate.

Institutional Review Board (IRB): A board designed to oversee the research process in order to protect participant safety. Made up of researchers, ethicists, and lay people from the community, the board must review the trial protocols and the informed consent forms participants sign.

Pharmacology: The science that deals with the effect of drugs on living organisms.

Phase 1 Trial: Small groups of people are treated with a certain dose of a new agent that has already been extensively studied in the laboratory. During the trial, the dose is usually increased group by group in order to determine a safe and appropriate dose to use in a phase 2 trial.

Phase 2 Trial: Phase 2 trials continue to test the safety of the new agent and begin to evaluate how well it works for a specific condition. In these trials, the new agent is given to groups of people using the dosage found to be safe in phase 1 trials.

Phase 3 Trial: Phase 3 studies are designed to answer research questions across the disease continuum. Phase 3 trials usually have hundreds to thousands of participants, in order to find out if there are true differences in the effectiveness of the treatment being tested.

Phase 4 Trial: Phase 4 trials are used to evaluate the long-term safety and effectiveness of a treatment. Less common than phase 1, 2, and 3 trials, phase 4 trials take place after the new treatment has been approved for standard use.

Placebo Controlled Study: A method of investigation of drugs in which an inactive substance (the placebo) is given to one group of participants, while the drug being tested is given to another group. The results obtained in the two groups are then compared to see if the investigational treatment is more effective in treating the condition.

Placebo Effect: A physical or emotional change, occurring after a substance is taken.

Placebo: A treatment, often a drug, designed to look like the investigational drug but that doesn't contain any active ingredient. Some people call a placebo a "sugar pill."

Protocol: A written plan that acts as a "recipe" for conducting a clinical trial. The protocol explains what a trial will do, how it will be carried out, and why each part of the trial is necessary.

Quality of Life: The overall enjoyment of life. Many clinical trials measure aspects of an individual's sense of well-being and ability to perform various tasks to assess the effects of treatment on the quality of life.

Randomization: A method used to prevent bias in research. A computer generates treatment assignments, and participants have an equal chance to be assigned to one of two or more groups (e.g., the control group or the investigational group).

Risk: The probability of an event occurring during a specified period of time.

Safety: No drug is completely safe or lacking the potential for side effects.

Side Effects: Any undesired actions or effects or a drug or treatment. Experimental drugs must be evaluated for both immediate and long-term side effects.

Standards of Care: Treatment regimen or medical management based on state of the art participant care.

Study Endpoint: A primary or secondary outcome used to judge the effectiveness of a treatment.

Notes

Notes

Notes

www.ingramcontent.com/pod-product-compliance
Lightning Source LLC
Chambersburg PA
CBHW032015190326
41520CB00007B/485